Overcoming the Fear of Flying - **A Pilot's Perspective**

OVERCOMING THE FEAR OF FLYING

A PILOT'S PERSPECTIVE

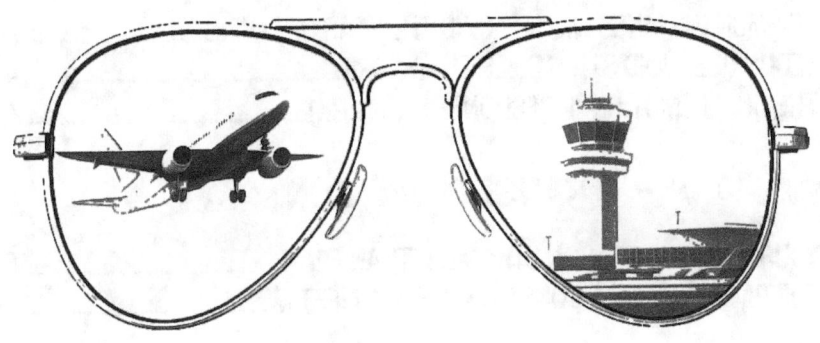

CAPTAIN
RON BENGOECHEA

CONTENTS

OVERCOMING THE FEAR OF FLYING

A PILOT'S PERSPECTIVE

Captain Ron Bengoechea

Pre-Flight Checklist

☐ <u>Boarding Completed</u>

☐ <u>Understand Fear</u>

☐ <u>See Through the Eyes of a Pilot</u>

☐ <u>Take Back Control</u>

☐ <u>Transform Fear into Confidence</u>

ADDITIONAL TOOLS ONBOARD

? FAQ: Real Questions from Passengers

🕐 10-Minute Pre-Flight Routine

🧠 Emotional Response Kit (QERK)

📋 Calm Scripts for Flight

INTRODUCTION

WHY YOU'RE HERE, AND WHY THIS BOOK MATTERS

One in three passengers feels anxious about flying. Maybe you're one of them. Maybe just reading those words makes your heart rate rise. If so, you're in the right place.

Flying anxiety is more common than you think. Millions of people struggle with it every year, yet very few talk about it openly. They keep it inside, hiding it from friends, family, even from themselves. But here's the truth: you're not broken, and you're not alone.

I've been a professional pilot for more than two decades. I've flown thousands of hours across continents and oceans, through turbulence, thunderstorms, and midnight skies. I've also seen passengers at their most vulnerable: trembling hands, shallow breathing, eyes glued to the seatbelt sign. I know how real this fear feels.

This is not my first book—it's part of my mission to help you change your story with flying. Not through theory or clichés, but through clear explanations, practical strategies, and small wins you can apply immediately. You don't need to read this book cover to cover before your next flight to feel a difference—you'll start noticing changes as early as the first chapters.

HERE'S THE KEY IDEA

Fear isn't the enemy. The story your brain tells about flying is.

Inside your mind lives a "Hollywood scriptwriter," always on call, ready to turn a harmless bump into a disaster movie. But you also have an inner captain—calm, rational, capable of leading you safely through turbulence, both in the sky and in your thoughts. This book will train that captain to take command.

By the end, you'll understand:

↳ •Why your brain reacts the way it does on airplanes.

↳ •How to stop catastrophic "What if...?" thoughts before they spiral.

↳ •How to use simple, proven techniques to calm your body and mind in real time.

↳ •How to replace limiting beliefs with empowering ones, so flying becomes not just bearable, but even freeing.

This isn't about eliminating fear entirely. It's about transforming it—so you regain choice, freedom, and control.

So, let's begin. Fasten your seatbelt, not because you're in danger, but because we're about to take off on a journey that will change the way you see flying forever.

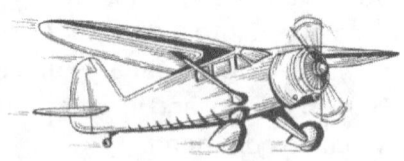

Pre-Flight Checklist

☑ Boarding Completed

☐ Understand Fear

☐ See Through the Eyes of a Pilot

☐ Take Back Control

☐ Transform Fear into Confidence

ADDITIONAL TOOLS ONBOARD

? FAQ: Real Questions from Passengers
🕐 10-Minute Pre-Flight Routine
🧠 Emotional Response Kit (QERK)
📜 Calm Scripts for Flight

PART I
UNDERSTANDING FEAR

CHAPTER 1

THE HIDDEN ENEMY: WHY FEAR OF FLYING EXISTS

You're not alone. The very fact that you're holding this book shows something important: you've already taken the bravest step—facing your fear instead of running from it.

Think about it: before every flight, pilots sit down and carefully plan the journey. In the same way, this first chapter is our flight plan. We're going to explore what really happens in your brain when fear takes control. Understanding is the beginning of freedom.

Let me start with a story that has been told for centuries in India.

In a small village, there lived a saint deeply loved by his people. When news spread that a smallpox epidemic was approaching, fear gripped every home. The saint, moved by compassion, entered into deep meditation and invoked the spirit of smallpox itself. When the spirit appeared, the saint pleaded for mercy. The spirit agreed: it would take only three lives and then leave the village.

That night, three villagers died. Saddened but grateful, the people accepted the loss, believing the danger had passed. Yet in the following nights, more and more villagers perished—not from the disease, but from terror. Panic spread faster than the sickness itself.

Distressed, the saint called upon the spirit again: 'You promised to take only three lives. Why are so many more dying?'

The spirit replied: 'I kept my promise. I only took three. The rest have been claimed by fear. It is fear that kills them, not me.'

This story, shared by Paramahansa Yogananda in Autobiography of a Yogi, reminds us of the destructive power of fear. Often, it is not the threat itself, but our own fear of it, that proves most deadly.

That's the power of fear—it can be more destructive than the threat itself.

And that's exactly what happens with the fear of flying. Flying is statistically the safest form of travel, yet fear convinces many that stepping onto a plane is risking their life. The danger is not the airplane—it's the story fear whispers in your mind.

THE BRAIN'S ALARM SYSTEM

To understand this better, let's look inside your own control tower: your brain.

There's a small structure called the amygdala—your internal alarm system. When it senses danger, it fires off signals that release adrenaline and cortisol. Your heart races, your breathing accelerates, and your muscles tense. This is the fight-or-flight response.

In the jungle, this saved our ancestors from lions. But your amygdala doesn't know the difference between a lion and turbulence at 35,000 feet. For the amygdala, both are threats.

Here's an example from my own career as a pilot. Years ago, when I was teaching the electrical systems of the DC-9, I discovered that the best way to keep other pilots awake in class was to surprise them. Instead of boring slides, I'd ask: "What is alternating current?" Everyone knew it powered their homes, but nobody could explain it clearly. Immediately, curiosity snapped them awake.

The amygdala works in the same way: it reacts strongly to anything uncommon or unfamiliar. A sudden sound during takeoff? Your brain screams, "What's this?!" even if it's completely normal. That's why understanding what happens on a plane—through education and clarity—is such a powerful antidote.

YOUR INNER HOLLYWOOD SCRIPTWRITER

But the amygdala is only half the story. There's another character in your mind: the executive function—your inner captain. Think of it as the captain of your flight. It works in three simple steps: analyze the situation, make a plan, and commit to it.

When your inner captain works well, it calms the amygdala. Imagine you hear an unusual noise during takeoff.

1. Analyze: Your captain-brain compares it to past experiences— "I've heard similar sounds before, it's probably the landing gear retracting."

2. Plan: It prepares a response—"Even if it happens again, it's not a danger signal."

3. Commit: Finally, it decides—"Everything is under control."

And with that, the amygdala relaxes.

But when your inner captain fails—when knowledge and commitment are missing—the inner Hollywood scriptwriter takes over. Suddenly, a harmless sound becomes the opening scene of a disaster movie: "What if the engine fails? What if we crash? What if I can't escape?" This is called anticipatory anxiety—your mind spinning "what if" stories about a future that isn't happening.

Here's how I like to picture it: your brain is a ship caught in a storm. The anxious thoughts are the waves crashing against the hull. But at the helm is an experienced captain. If the captain panics, the ship is lost. If the captain holds steady, the ship stays on course.

That captain is you—once you learn how to take control of your thoughts.

A PRACTICAL EXERCISE FOR YOU

Right now, grab a notebook or your phone and write down one common "What if...?" thought you have about flying.

For example:

- "What if the turbulence makes the plane fall?"

Then answer it with logic, as your captain-brain would:

- "Turbulence is uncomfortable but not dangerous. Airplanes are designed for it, and pilots are trained to handle it."

Now it's your turn. Write down two or three of your own "What if...?" thoughts. For each one, challenge it with facts or logic. Remember, your goal isn't to deny the fear but to put it in perspective.

Congratulations—you've just practiced the first step of replacing fear with truth. Do this often, and you'll start training your mind to switch from anxious storytelling to calm reasoning—just like a captain keeping the ship steady in rough seas.

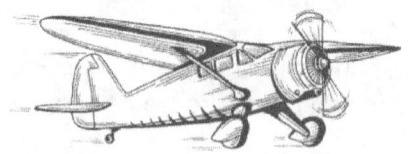

CHAPTER 2

THE SCRIPTWRITER IN YOUR MIND

When you sit on a plane and your heart begins to race before the engines even start, it isn't the aircraft that's creating danger—it's your own inner "Hollywood scriptwriter." This part of your mind takes the smallest detail—a sound, a bump, a thought—and turns it into a full-blown disaster movie.

Understanding this scriptwriter is key, because until you see how it works, you'll always believe its stories. And those stories feel real, even when they're pure fiction.

HOW ANXIETY CREATES DISASTER MOVIES

Anxiety loves to play director. It starts with a "what if...?"

- ↳ • What if the turbulence gets worse?
- ↳ • What if that noise means something is broken?
- ↳ • What if I panic in front of everyone?

Each "what if" is like the opening scene of a thriller, and your mind quickly fills in the rest—imaginary failures, dramatic crashes, terrible outcomes. Soon, you're watching a film inside your head that feels more convincing than reality itself.

The truth? These movies are just anxiety's way of keeping you hooked. They are not predictions. They are mental fiction.

ANTICIPATORY THOUGHTS VS. REALITY

Fear of flying rarely strikes in the moment. It begins days, weeks, even months before the trip. This is anticipatory anxiety—the endless rehearsal of everything that might go wrong.

The Danish philosopher Søren Kierkegaard once described anxiety as "the dizziness of freedom"—a fear that arises not from what is happening, but from imagining what could happen. In flying, this shows up as a constant inner rehearsal of "what if" scenarios that never actually take place.

OVERCOMING THE FEAR OF FLYING — A PILOT'S PERSPECTIVE

But here's the critical distinction:

- o Anticipatory thoughts are symptoms of nervousness.
- o Reality is what actually happens in flight.

I know this mechanism well, even beyond the cockpit. For me, it often shows up in everyday situations. For example, before giving a talk to a large audience or while teaching, my mind sometimes races ahead, imagining escape routes or worst-case scenarios: "What if I forget what to say? What if I freeze?"

In reality, none of those things happen—but the script in my head feels so real that my body reacts as if it were true. That's the same mechanism passengers experience when a flight is approaching. The mind writes a disaster script long before the first engine turns on.

SHORT STORY OF A PASSENGER WHO DIDN'T READ THIS BOOK

Let me give you a real example from the cockpit. Over the years, I've witnessed countless reactions from passengers, and this one illustrates the power of fear perfectly.

A passenger boarded a flight to Paris. As the plane accelerated and the landing gear retracted, a small vibration was felt—a sound I had heard thousands of times and knew was perfectly normal.

But for this passenger, the amygdala—the brain's alarm center—fired instantly: Danger!

Now the scriptwriter took over. Within seconds, the passenger's mind created a disaster movie:

↳ •What if the gear is broken?

↳ •What if the plane can't land?

↳ •What if we crash?

Their heart raced, their palms sweated, and panic took hold.

Meanwhile, the rest of the passengers sat calmly—some reading, some already dozing off. The only difference? They didn't let their inner scriptwriter take control.

That's how powerful these internal movies can be: one sound, two completely different realities.

REFRAMING THE SCRIPT: FROM FEAR TO FACTS

The good news is that you don't have to believe every disaster movie your mind plays. You can catch the scriptwriter in the act—and even rewrite the story. Here's how:

1. **CATCH THE "WHAT IF"**

    ↳ Every anxious thought starts with those two words: "What if...?" The moment you hear it in your mind, pause. Label it: "This is not reality, this is my scriptwriter talking." Simply naming it gives you distance and stops the automatic spiral before it takes over.

2. **SWAP FICTION FOR FACTS**

    ↳ Now bring in logic. Remind yourself: airplanes are designed to handle turbulence, noises are part of normal operation, and pilots train thousands of hours for emergencies that almost never happen. Facts don't erase fear instantly, but they weaken the scriptwriter's grip by bringing you back to what is real, not imagined.

3. **REDIRECT THE STORY**

    ↳ Finally, give your mind a new script. Instead of imagining disaster, ask: "What is the most likely thing happening right now?" 99% of the time, the answer will be: "Nothing unusual. Just another safe flight." By doing this, you're not only calming your amygdala—you're training your brain to replace fear with truth, over and over again.

A PILOT'S LESSON FROM THE CLASSROOM

Early in my career, I became an instructor on the DC-9, responsible for teaching other pilots about aircraft systems. One of my favorite subjects was the electrical system.

Now, most expected a boring, step-by-step technical class. But I learned that if you teach like that, the brain shuts down. Students' minds wander, and they start writing their own scripts—usually of boredom or frustration.

So I did something different. I would ask unexpected questions, create unusual scenarios, and break the monotony. Suddenly, those same pilots who were bracing themselves for hours of boredom were engaged, curious, even excited.

Why? Because their script had changed. Instead of a dull story of "another systems class," they were now in an unexpected, stimulating experience that kept them alert and motivated.

And that's exactly how fear of flying works. The "classroom" is your flight. If you let your mind play the same old script—"this is going to be awful, I won't be able to handle it"—then the experience becomes boring at best and terrifying at worst. But when you consciously change the script, the experience itself changes. A flight can shift from being a long chain of "what ifs" into an opportunity: a chance to travel, to reunite with family, to discover something new.

The principle is simple but powerful: change the script, and you change the experience.

PRACTICAL EXERCISE: "REWRITE THE SCENE"

Write down one anxious thought you often have about flying.

Example: "What if the turbulence gets so bad the plane breaks apart?"

Next to it, write a grounded fact that counters the fear. For example:

"Airplanes are tested to withstand forces far stronger than turbulence, and pilots are trained to handle it as a normal part of flying."

Now read that fact three times out loud. Don't just repeat the words—pay attention to how your body reacts. Most people notice their breathing slows, their shoulders drop, and their mind feels steadier.

The next time your scriptwriter tries to play a disaster movie, you'll already have a rewritten script ready—one based on truth, not fear.

KEY TAKEAWAY

Fear of flying isn't born in the engines, the wings, or the sky—it's born in the stories your mind creates. By learning to see your inner scriptwriter at work, you take back the director's chair. From this point on, the only movie you allow to play is the one grounded in facts, not fear.

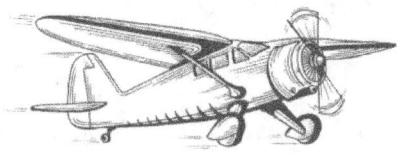

CHAPTER 3

FEAR, BELIEFS, AND THE STORIES WE TELL OURSELVES

Fear doesn't just live in the amygdala or in the "Hollywood movies" your mind creates. It also hides in the quiet background of your beliefs—the stories you've been telling yourself for years.

If you believe "flying is dangerous," no amount of statistics will calm you down. If you believe "I'm not strong enough to handle turbulence," you'll panic at the first bump. Beliefs shape perception, and perception becomes reality.

The good news? Beliefs aren't permanent. They can be rewritten, just like the script in your mind.

LIMITING VS. EMPOWERING BELIEFS

Think of beliefs as the lenses on your glasses. If the lens is scratched, dirty, or tinted the wrong way, the world looks distorted. The objects in front of you haven't changed, but your perception of them has. You might misinterpret shadows as obstacles or colors as signals of danger, simply because of the way you're looking through the lens.

It's the same with flying. When your beliefs are limiting, they filter reality in a way that makes every sound, movement, or sensation feel threatening.

Limiting beliefs:

o "I can't control my fear."

o "If I panic, something terrible will happen."

o "Flying is unnatural; we don't belong in the sky."

These beliefs act like invisible anchors, holding you back and making every flight a struggle.

But you can change the lens. By shifting beliefs, the very same flight can be experienced with curiosity, calm, or even gratitude.

Empowering beliefs:

- o "Fear is just a signal, not a prophecy."

- o "I can use tools to calm myself."

- o "Flying connects me with the people and places I love."

These beliefs lift you up, creating freedom instead of restriction. The first step is simply learning to notice which set of lenses you're wearing—distorted ones that keep you trapped, or clear ones that allow you to see flying for what it truly is.

STORY: TWO PASSENGERS, ONE FLIGHT

I've seen this countless times from the cockpit. Two passengers can be sitting just a few rows apart on the exact same flight. The plane hits a pocket of turbulence.

One passenger grips the armrest, heart racing, convinced that every bump is a sign of danger. Their belief is: "This isn't normal, we're in trouble."

Meanwhile, the other passenger barely looks up from their book, maybe even smiles and adjusts their seatbelt. Their belief is: "Turbulence is part of flying, nothing unusual."

The reality is identical—the same plane, the same turbulence, the same sky. What changes is not the fact, but the belief. And that single difference creates two completely different experiences: one of panic, the other of calm.

That's exactly how fear of flying works. The facts don't change— planes are safe, pilots are trained—but your beliefs about them make all the difference.

HOW BELIEFS SHAPE PERCEPTION

Your beliefs act like filters.

↳ •If you believe a strange sound means danger, you'll tense up immediately.

↳ •If you believe a sound is part of normal operation, you'll barely notice it.

The difference is not reality—it's the story you attach to reality.

This is why two passengers can sit side by side on the same flight: one sweating and panicked, the other reading a book peacefully. They aren't living in the same "outer" reality. They're living in different "inner" realities shaped by their beliefs.

THE THRIVE METHOD: TRANSFORMING BELIEFS STEP BY STEP

The THRIVE Method is more than an acronym—it's a mental checklist.

The original version was designed to help people transform limiting beliefs into empowering ones. I've adapted it to the world of flying, where fear can grow out of a single "what if" thought. Here's how both versions connect, so you get the best of each.

1.   T – TARGET THE BELIEF (OR THINK)

Original: Think—recognize the limiting thought. You can't change what you don't notice.

Applied: Target—pinpoint the exact fear fueling your anxiety.

Example: "If turbulence gets bad, the plane might break."

Naming the belief clearly is like putting it under a spotlight—suddenly it loses some of its power.

2.   H – HIGHLIGHT THE EVIDENCE (OR HALT)

Original: Halt—pause and question whether the thought is actually true.

Applied: Highlight—weigh the evidence for and against the fear.

Look at facts: planes are engineered to withstand far more stress than turbulence, and pilots train thousands of hours for every scenario.

The moment you shine a light on reality, fear begins to shrink.

3.   R – REPLACE WITH FACTS

Original: Replace—swap the limiting belief for an empowering one.

Applied: Do the same, but in the language of flying.

Example: Change "Turbulence means danger" to "Turbulence is uncomfortable but safe. Pilots handle it every day."

This shift is the turning point: fear gives way to truth.

4.   I – INTEGRATE IT DAILY (OR INGRAIN)

Original: Ingrain—embed the new belief through repetition.

Applied: Integrate—practice before boarding, during flight, even at home. Beliefs are like muscles: they strengthen with use.

The more you repeat your new script, the faster it becomes automatic.

5.   V – VISUALIZE THE NEW REALITY (OR VALIDATE)

Original: Validate—test and confirm that the new belief is working.

Applied: Visualize—see yourself calm during turbulence, breathing steadily, staying present. Mental rehearsal is powerful: your brain starts believing what it sees.

Validation comes when reality matches the picture you've been practicing.

6.   E – EVALUATE PROGRESS (OR ENFORCE)

Original: Enforce—repeat the process to make it stick.

Applied: Evaluate—after each flight, ask: "How did my new belief help me?" Every reflection reinforces the change, and every small win builds confidence for the next journey.

EXERCISE: BELIEF REFRAME JOURNAL

Tonight, set aside just 10 minutes. Write down three beliefs you have about flying. For each belief, ask yourself:

o   Is this belief limiting me or empowering me?

o   What story am I attaching to it? (For example: "If I panic, I'll lose control.")

o   How could I rewrite it using the THRIVE Method?

Example:

o   Limiting belief: "Turbulence means the plane is in danger."

o   Reframed with THRIVE: "Turbulence is uncomfortable but safe. Planes are designed for it, and pilots are trained to handle it."

Do this daily for a week. You'll begin to notice a shift: the next time you step onto a plane, those old anchors of fear will feel lighter, and your new beliefs will start to carry you forward with confidence.

KEY TAKEAWAY

Fear isn't just about alarms in your brain or nervous thoughts—it's about the stories you believe. The good news is: stories can be rewritten.

By spotting limiting beliefs and transforming them into empowering ones, you take back the captain's seat of your mind.

Flying then becomes more than a way to travel—it becomes your personal training ground for courage, a chance to practice rewriting the stories that shape not just your flights, but your life.

Pre-Flight Checklist

☑ Boarding Completed

☑ Understand Fear

☐ See Through the Eyes of a Pilot

☐ Take Back Control

☐ Transform Fear into Confidence

ADDITIONAL TOOLS ONBOARD

? FAQ: Real Questions from Passengers

🕐 10-Minute Pre-Flight Routine

🧠 Emotional Response Kit (QERK)

📋 Calm Scripts for Flight

PART II

A PILOT'S PERSPECTIVE

CHAPTER 4

FROM PILOT TO PASSENGER: SEEING THROUGH MY EYES

When you step onto an airplane as a passenger, you see seats, windows, and cabin crew. When I step onto an airplane as a pilot, I see something completely different: a finely tuned machine designed to protect you in every possible scenario.

One of the fastest ways to calm fear is to borrow my eyes—to see what I see when I look at an aircraft. Because the truth is this: airplanes are built to be safe. Not "safe enough," but layers upon layers of safety, far beyond what most people imagine.

WHY AIRPLANES ARE DESIGNED TO BE SAFE

Every commercial aircraft must prove, through thousands of hours of tests, that it can keep flying even if major systems fail. Redundancy is the golden rule: there are always backups.

Let me give you an example from my time flying Boeing. During training, we practiced what's called an engine-out scenario— simulating the loss of an engine right after takeoff. Most passengers imagine this would be catastrophic. But in reality, the aircraft continues climbing, the systems adapt, and the pilots calmly follow the procedure.

I've practiced this scenario countless times in the simulator—and even once in real life. The airplane performed exactly as designed: stable, reliable, and determined to keep us safe.

That's the real character of modern airplanes. They're not fragile; they're stubborn survivors.

WHAT HAPPENS DURING A FLIGHT (STEP BY STEP)

Fear thrives in the unknown. So let's walk through the entire journey together, phase by phase. I'll show you what you hear or feel in your seat—and what's really happening in the cockpit. Once you know the script, flying stops being a mystery and becomes just another routine.

1.   ENGINE START-UP

o What you hear: a whirring, followed by a deep "whoosh."

o What's happening: the auxiliary power unit (a small engine in the tail) brings the big engines to life. The sound grows from a soft growl to a steady hum.

o Reassurance: it may sound dramatic, but this is simply the airplane waking up—perfectly normal.

2.   TAXI

o What you feel: gentle turns, sometimes a bump or vibration over seams in the pavement.

o What's happening: the pilots steer the airplane with a small nose wheel, just like a car, guided by ground control.

o Reassurance: these little jolts don't mean trouble—they're just the "road bumps" of the airport.

3.   TAKEOFF

o What you hear: engines roar, the airplane accelerates fast, sometimes with vibrations.

o What's happening: we apply maximum thrust to lift the aircraft. Vibrations are just raw power at work. At rotation speed, the nose rises, and the airplane lifts smoothly into the sky.

o Reassurance: that powerful push you feel is exactly what we want—it means your journey has truly begun.

4.   CLIMB

o What you notice: a strong upward angle, and then suddenly the engines get quieter.

o What's happening: once safely airborne, we reduce thrust to climb power. The sudden quiet often surprises passengers, but it's exactly what should happen.

o Reassurance: less noise doesn't mean less safety—it's the sound of efficiency.

5.   CRUISE

o What you feel: smooth, stable flight, sometimes gentle turbulence.

o What's happening: the autopilot takes over, flying with precision measured in centimeters. Meanwhile, pilots monitor weather, systems, and communications.

o Reassurance: this is the calm heart of the journey. Even when turbulence appears, the airplane is built to handle it with ease.

6.   DESCENT

o What you hear: a low rumble, hisses, or thumps.

o What's happening: flaps extend to give the wings more lift at slower speeds; the cabin pressure adjusts gradually to match the ground.

o Reassurance: these noises are the airplane carefully preparing for a safe landing.

7.   LANDING

o What you hear: the landing gear lowering with a heavy clunk, more airflow noise, then a firm touchdown followed by reverse thrust (a loud roar).

o What's happening: the gear locks into place, the tires meet the runway, and reverse thrust slows the plane.

o Reassurance: every sound here signals control—the airplane is simply coming to a safe stop.

Every phase has its own soundtrack. Once you know what's happening, you realize flying isn't an unknown threat—it's a carefully choreographed routine, repeated thousands of times every day around the world.

TURBULENCE, STRANGE NOISES, AND WHY THEY'RE HARMLESS

If there's one thing that makes passengers grip the armrest tighter, it's turbulence. The bumps, the seatbelt sign, the coffee that suddenly shakes—it feels like the airplane is losing control. But here's the truth: turbulence is uncomfortable, not dangerous.

WHY TURBULENCE FEELS WORSE THAN IT IS

Your brain interprets sudden movements as danger. The amygdala doesn't know the difference between a lion in the jungle and a bump of air at 35,000 feet. Add to this the fact that airplanes move fast—so even small shifts feel dramatic—and you get the perfect recipe for panic.

But here's the technical reality: airplanes are built to withstand far more than turbulence. Wings flex, fuselages bend, engines generate more power than any wind current in the sky. What feels unstable to you is well within the design limits of the aircraft.

A STORY FROM THE COCKPIT

I once sat next to a passenger during a flight when we hit some light to moderate turbulence. He immediately tensed, eyes on the seatbelt sign that had just lit up.

I smiled and told him: "Actually, I'm glad this happened—it gives us a chance to talk about turbulence."

I explained that we pilots sometimes joke about the seatbelt sign as the "lawyer light." Why? Because it protects the airline in case someone decides to stand up, gets bumped, and hurts themselves. The light doesn't mean danger for the plane—it just means: "Please sit down and buckle up, so you don't get hurt."

Still, he looked skeptical. So I asked him:

"Have you ever been on a boat during rough seas?"

"Yes," he replied.

"Would you walk around the bow of the boat in the middle of those waves?"

"Of course not," he said.

"That's exactly what turbulence is. The plane is safe, but it's not the right time to be walking around."

To make it more real, I asked him to sip his drink while the turbulence continued. He did. "See? No problem," I said. "Now think of drinking water in a car going over a bumpy road. Which is harder?" He laughed—he knew the answer.

Finally, I gave him one of my favorite comparisons:

"Imagine a toy airplane inside a block of gelatin. Shake the gelatin, and the airplane moves with it. But it never falls out, never loses its place. That's turbulence. The airplane is held by the air just as securely as that toy inside the gelatin."

His shoulders relaxed. By the end of the flight, he admitted that he had forgotten about the turbulence entirely—proof that attention and perspective change the experience.

TYPES OF TURBULENCE

o Thermal Turbulence: caused by hot air rising from the ground, especially on warm days. To passengers, it feels like sharp bumps at lower altitudes or during climb. Perfectly normal.

o Cloud Turbulence: formed inside clouds by temperature differences. It can look dramatic, but the air currents are smooth and predictable.

o Clear Air Turbulence (CAT): invisible, found where fast- and slow-moving air meet. Modern autopilots and aircraft handle this gently, without stress on the airplane.

INTENSITY LEVELS

o Light: gentle bumps, like driving over a slightly uneven road. Annoying maybe, but barely noticeable for the airplane.

o Moderate: more obvious shaking—you'll feel it, but the plane itself remains completely stable and under control. Pilots handle this every day.

o Severe: can feel intense and uncomfortable, yet it's never dangerous. Think of the gelatin analogy: the plane wiggles inside the air, but it doesn't "fall." The structure and systems are built to withstand far more than what passengers ever experience.

HOW PILOTS MANAGE IT

Pilots are never passive. We receive turbulence reports from aircraft ahead of us, adjust altitude, or change course to minimize discomfort. Passenger comfort matters, and avoiding bumps when possible is part of our daily job.

STRANGE NOISES

Turbulence isn't the only trigger. Strange noises during flight—landing gear retracting, flaps moving, engines adjusting—can startle passengers. But every sound has a purpose. Airplanes are machines in constant motion, and those noises are the sound of systems working as designed.

When you hear a thump or a whir, remember: for the pilots in the cockpit, it's business as usual. If it were anything else, you'd know immediately from their calm voices and the steady progress of the flight.

REAL STORIES FROM THE COCKPIT

One night, I was flying across the Intertropical Convergence Zone— the belt near the equator where warm, humid air masses collide and rise, creating some of the most powerful thunderstorms on Earth. Pilots call it the "ITCZ," and it's a place where lightning shows and turbulence are simply part of the scenery.

That night over Africa, flying east to west, flashes of lightning lit up the sky while turbulence rocked the airplane. I could sense passenger anxiety, but inside the cockpit, we stayed calm. Our weather radar painted the storm cells clearly, allowing us to navigate safely around them. The airplane remained steady, doing exactly what it was designed to do.

When we landed and I was saying goodbye to the passengers, a lady told me, "I thought we were in real danger." I explained how the aircraft is built to handle those conditions, and how radar helps us avoid the strongest areas. Her fear turned into amazement once she understood the reality behind the experience.

And that reaction is more common than you might think. Many fears in flying don't come from real danger, but from the unfamiliar: loud sounds, sudden movements, or the sight of a storm outside the window. What feels alarming to a passenger often means something completely routine to a pilot.

Another time, a passenger panicked at the loud thud of the landing gear coming down. For us pilots, that sound is reassuring—it means everything is working exactly as it should. In fact, after years of flying, you barely notice it anymore. It's not that you don't hear it—it's that your focus is elsewhere, on the cockpit indications confirming that the gear is locked and down. That solid "clunk" is nothing more than the system doing its job, a routine confirmation that the airplane is ready to land safely.

After the flight, I explained this to him, and he laughed nervously: "So that sound that scared me is actually a good thing?" Exactly. Every sound in an airplane has a meaning. And once you understand what those sounds mean, fear begins to lose its grip.

KEY TAKEAWAY

Airplanes are not fragile—they're overbuilt, overtested, and constantly monitored. Every bump, every noise, every shake has a purpose.

So when turbulence hits or a strange sound echoes through the cabin, remind yourself:

"This is the airplane doing its job. The pilots expect this. I am safe."

Once you learn to see flying through a pilot's eyes, fear loses its script—and you regain your freedom to travel with confidence.

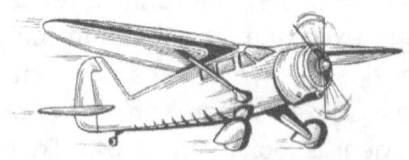

CHAPTER 5

KNOWLEDGE IS CALM: TECHNICAL INSIGHTS FOR PASSENGERS

One of the most powerful antidotes to fear is knowledge. Fear thrives in the shadows, where we don't understand what's happening. But the moment we turn on the light of clarity, the fear loses its power. In this chapter, I'll walk you through some of the most common concerns passengers have—automation, pressurization, emergencies, ocean crossings, mechanical failures—and show you, from my perspective as a pilot, why each of these is safe and manageable.

THE ROLE OF AUTOPILOT AND MODERN TECHNOLOGY

Once, while sitting with a passenger, the cockpit door opened and the captain stepped out. My seatmate's eyes widened: "Who's flying the plane now?"

I smiled: "The best pilot of all, but the one who earns the least... the autopilot."

He looked puzzled, so I explained.

The autopilot is one of the greatest achievements of modern aviation. It flies with incredible precision—making constant adjustments, smoother than any human could maintain for hours. It doesn't replace the pilots; it supports them. One pilot always stays at the controls, monitoring the systems, ready to intervene instantly. Automation reduces workload, prevents fatigue, and adds redundancy.

Far from being a weakness, it's one of aviation's greatest strengths. Knowing this helped my seatmate relax—he realized the airplane is never left unattended. It's always under the combined watch of humans and machines.

PRESSURIZATION AND OXYGEN MASKS EXPLAINED SIMPLY

Later, my seatmate mentioned that his ears felt blocked. I explained why: as we climb or descend, the air pressure changes. The cabin is pressurized to keep us comfortable, but your body sometimes needs a moment to adjust. Yawning or chewing gum helps equalize the pressure in your ears.

I told him: "Think of the cabin as a balloon. It's carefully regulated, never overinflated. Outflow valves constantly adjust to keep everything balanced."

Without pressurization, flying at 35,000 feet would feel like being on top of a very high mountain—thin air, difficult to breathe. Pressurization keeps the cabin feeling like you're at around 6,000–8,000 feet, which is perfectly safe.

He then asked about failures. I reassured him: in my 25 years of flying, I've never faced a real pressurization emergency. But we train for it constantly in simulators. If it ever happens, the procedure is straightforward: we simply descend quickly—within about 10 minutes or even less—to a safe, breathable altitude. It's not a "falling out of the sky" scenario—it's a calm, controlled maneuver that every pilot is prepared for.

That knowledge alone made him sigh in relief.

EMERGENCY PROCEDURES: WHY WE TRAIN FOR THE IMPOSSIBLE

In 25 years of flying, with more than 12,000 flight hours, I've only faced one situation that required shutting down an engine in flight. It happened on a DC-9-30, flying from the Dominican Republic to Curaçao, when the oil quantity on one engine suddenly dropped. The correct procedure was a precautionary shutdown.

Flying with one engine may sound alarming, but airplanes are designed for it. In fact, most passengers on that flight wouldn't have noticed anything if we hadn't informed them. The airplane remained stable, safe, and fully capable of reaching our destination.

The reason we shut it down was simple: that engine had lost its oil. On an older aircraft like the DC-9, this required immediate action to prevent damage. The DC-9 was a reliable airplane, but its systems were nowhere near as advanced as today's jets.

Years later, I had the privilege of flying the Dreamliner, the Boeing 787. On that aircraft, equipped with Rolls-Royce engines, the same condition—a loss of oil—would not necessarily require shutting the engine down. The technology is so advanced that the engine can continue operating safely while multiple systems monitor and manage the situation automatically.

This contrast shows how far aviation has evolved. What once required decisive manual action is now managed seamlessly by modern systems, always with safety as the priority.

The truth is: emergencies in aviation are extremely rare, but preparation is constant. That's why flying remains the safest way to travel.

FLYING OVER OCEANS, NIGHT FLIGHTS, AND THE UN-KNOWN

One day, while flying as a passenger across the Bay of Biscay, the person sitting next to me looked down at the endless water and asked: 'How do you know where you're going when there's nothing to see?

It's a great question. For those who fear flying, the unknown often feels like danger. But here's the reality: airplanes don't depend on what the eye can see. We navigate using advanced systems—satellites, GPS, and multiple backups.

I explained it this way: think of your car's GPS, but imagine it far more accurate and reliable. Airplanes connect to a global network of satellites and ground stations that track our exact position within a few meters, constantly cross-checking each other.

That means even in the middle of the ocean, or under a pitch-black night sky with no visible landmarks, the airplane always knows exactly where it is—often with more precision than the GPS in your car.

Over the ocean, over land, by day or by night—it makes no difference. Navigation is never guesswork. We always know where we are.

FEAR OF MECHANICAL FAILURES & STRANGE SOUNDS

The fear of "something breaking" is one of the most common anxieties I hear. The truth is that airplanes undergo constant inspections and maintenance. Engines are extremely reliable, designed with layers of redundancy. If one engine fails (again, extremely rare), the aircraft continues flying safely with the other.

Noise is another common trigger. Many times during descent, passengers sitting near me have heard a humming or a sudden mechanical sound and looked nervous. I explain: "That's the hydraulic system moving the flaps and slats. They extend to give the wings more lift at lower speeds, so the airplane can land safely."

To make it clearer, I often ask: "What do you think airplanes are designed for—flying fast or flying slow?"

"Fast," they usually reply.

"Exactly. Airplanes are built to be both safe and efficient, and that means flying fast at cruising altitude—where they spend most of their time. But for takeoff and landing, we need to slow down, so we change the shape of the wing using flaps and slats. That's what you're hearing."

The look of relief on their faces always says it all. What sounded like danger was, in reality, the sound of safety.

PRACTICAL EXERCISE – FACT VS. FICTION LOG

Grab a notebook or a sheet of paper and create two columns.

Left column (Fiction): Write down three fears, doubts, or unsettling thoughts you've had during flights—for example, "the engines suddenly got quieter" or "the plane shook during turbulence."

Right column (Fact): Next to each one, write the factual explanation you've just learned in this chapter—for instance, "engines get quieter because we reduce power after takeoff—it's exactly what should happen."

o Step it up: After writing your list, read the "fact" column out loud, slowly, three times. Notice how your body feels calmer when your brain hears the truth, not just your imagination.

o Repeat before flying: Each time you fly, review your list and add new examples. Over time, your brain will automatically replace fiction with facts—and fear will lose its script.

KEY TAKEAWAY

Airplanes are not mysteries. They're carefully designed, rigorously tested, and constantly monitored machines operated by highly trained professionals. Every sound, every bump, every change you notice has a reason—and that reason is safety.

The more you understand, the calmer you'll feel. Knowledge doesn't just answer your questions—it silences your fears.

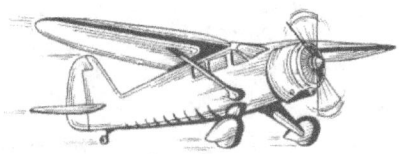

CAPTAIN RON BENGOECHEA

Pre-Flight Checklist

☑ <u>Boarding Completed</u>

☑ <u>Understand Fear</u>

☑ <u>See Through the Eyes of a Pilot</u>

☐ <u>Take Back Control</u>

☐ <u>Transform Fear into Confidence</u>

ADDITIONAL TOOLS ONBOARD

? FAQ: Real Questions from Passengers
🕐 10-Minute Pre-Flight Routine
🧠 Emotional Response Kit (QERK)
📜 Calm Scripts for Flight

PART III
TAKING BACK CONTROL

You already know how fear works. You've seen the cockpit through my eyes. Now it's time for the most important part: taking back control. In this section you'll train simple, practical responses so your mind stops running on autopilot and starts following your lead.

CHAPTER 6

COMMON MISTAKES WHEN FACING THE FEAR OF FLYING

Overcoming fear of flying is not about willpower. It's about strategy. Over the years, I've seen many passengers repeat the same mistakes again and again. The good news? Once you recognize them, you can avoid them.

Before I hand you the tools that will truly help you, let's look at the traps that keep fear alive. Over the years, I've seen many passengers repeat the same patterns—mistakes that seemed harmless but actually made their anxiety worse.

This chapter is your pre-flight safety check: avoid these errors, and you'll be ready to use the techniques in the next chapter with much more power.

MISTAKE 1: RELYING ON ALCOHOL OR PILLS WITHOUT CONTROL

A glass of wine or a pill may feel like a solution, but it's a trap. Alcohol dehydrates you, raises anxiety, and increases the sense of losing control. Medication, when prescribed by a doctor, can sometimes help—but it's not a magic cure. Fear isn't solved at the bottom of a glass.

MISTAKE 2: AVOIDING FLYING ALTOGETHER

It seems like a relief, but avoidance only strengthens fear. Each time you say "I won't fly," your brain learns that the only way to feel safe is to avoid. And so the fear grows stronger, not weaker.

MISTAKE 3: FEEDING YOUR FEAR WITH CATASTROPHIC INFORMATION

Some people search "plane crash" videos or binge disaster documentaries before a flight. That's like pouring fuel into the Hollywood scriptwriter in your mind. If you want information, look for real data from reliable sources—not sensationalist stories.

MISTAKE 4: EXPECTING FEAR TO DISAPPEAR OVERNIGHT

Many believe they'll step on a plane, try one technique, and suddenly be cured forever. That's not how it works. Fear fades with practice, flight by flight, step by step. Every flight is training—and progress is built gradually.

MISTAKE 5: SKIPPING PREPARATION BEFORE THE FLIGHT

Anxiety usually starts long before you reach the airport. If you don't practice your tools on the ground—breathing, visualization, anchors—it's harder to apply them in the air. Preparation on the ground = success in the sky.

MISTAKE 6: COMPARING YOURSELF TO OTHER PASSENGERS

"Everyone else looks calm, so I must be broken." False. Many people hide their anxiety. Comparison only adds pressure. Your journey is yours alone, and every small win counts.

MISTAKE 7: DEPENDING ONLY ON DISTRACTION

Movies, music, or games help, but if distraction is your only tool, you're just escaping. True freedom comes from combining distraction with conscious techniques that change how you react to fear.

MISTAKE 8: INTERPRETING EVERY SOUND OR MOVEMENT AS DANGER

A noise, a bump, or a moment of silence—and the alarm in your mind goes off. One of the biggest mistakes is assuming normal equals dangerous. The truth: these are everyday signs of flight. The key is to retrain your brain to see them as routine, not threats.

PRACTICAL KEY

Fear feeds on three roots:

↳ Avoidance.

↳ Wrong interpretations.

↳ Unrealistic expectations.

Cut these roots, and fear loses its power.

TECHNIQUES AND STRATEGIES THAT WORK

Fear of flying is not just in the airplane—it's in the mind. The thoughts, images, and sensations that arise before and during the flight are what make the experience overwhelming. The good news? Those thoughts and sensations can be trained, redirected, and calmed.

In this chapter, I'll share with you the exact techniques I've seen work, both with passengers and in my own professional journey as a pilot. They are simple, but powerful when practiced consistently.

AWARENESS OF THOUGHTS AND EMOTIONS

The first step in taking back control is awareness. Most of the time, anxious thoughts run in the background like a movie on autoplay:

↳ "What if something happens?"

↳ "What was that sound?"

↳ "I don't think I can handle this."

Your brain reacts as if these thoughts were real threats. But they are just that—thoughts.

Try this exercise: The next time you feel a wave of anxiety, don't fight it. Instead, label it. Say to yourself: "This is fear. This is my brain trying to protect me." By naming it, you create distance between yourself and the emotion.

Think of it like sitting in a cinema. You can watch the movie on the screen, but you're not inside it.

VISUALIZING YOUR CALM SELF

Your mind is powerful, and it doesn't distinguish much between what's real and what's imagined. That's why visualizing a calm flight is one of the most effective ways to reprogram your response.

Close your eyes and imagine:

- ↳ Sitting in your seat, breathing deeply, shoulders relaxed.
- ↳ Hearing the engines roar on takeoff and smiling, knowing this is just power doing its job.
- ↳ Feeling turbulence and saying to yourself: "The plane is doing exactly what it was built to do."

The more vividly you rehearse these images, the more natural they become when you are actually in the situation. Top athletes do this before competitions—so why not you, before your flight?

BREATHING, GROUNDING, AND FLOW TECHNIQUES

When fear takes over, your body reacts: shallow breathing, tense muscles, racing heart. The quickest way to calm it down is through the breath.

BOX BREATHING (4X4)

- ↳ Inhale through your nose for 4 seconds.
- ↳ Hold your breath for 4 seconds.
- ↳ Exhale slowly for 4 seconds.
- ↳ Hold again for 4 seconds.
- ↳ Repeat 4 times.

This simple pattern tells your nervous system: "It's safe to relax."

GROUNDING EXERCISE

Look around and name:

- 5 things you can see.
- 4 things you can touch.
- 3 things you can hear.
- 2 things you can smell.
- 1 thing you can taste.

This pulls your mind away from fear and into the present moment.

FLOW TECHNIQUE

Instead of resisting sensations (like turbulence), imagine yourself "flowing" with them. Let your body move naturally with the bumps, just as you would sway with waves on a boat. Resistance creates tension; flow creates calm.

QUICK PATTERNS (WHEN X → DO Y)

- When your heart races → Box Breathing 4×4.
- When "what if" thoughts appear → Label it: "That's my scriptwriter, not reality."
- When your body feels tight → Scan shoulders, jaw, and hands, then release.
- When scary images pop up → Replace them with your Calm Self visualization.

STEPPING OUTSIDE YOUR COMFORT ZONE GRADUALLY

Courage isn't the absence of fear—it's progress in small steps. You don't need to conquer your fear in one leap; you need to face it in layers.

Start with what feels manageable:

↳ Spend a few minutes at an airport just watching airplanes take off and land.

↳ Book a short flight—one hour or less. Practice your breathing and visualization during it.

↳ Gradually extend to longer flights, each time applying the techniques.

↳ Every successful step teaches your brain a new truth: "I can do this. I am safe."

PRACTICAL EXERCISE – YOUR CALM FLIGHT BLUEPRINT

1. List your fears. Write down three fears that usually come up before or during a flight.

2. Create your response. For each one, write a new explanation you'll practice.

    • Example:

        • Fear: "The engines got quieter."

        • Response: "That means we reduced thrust for climb— it's normal."

3. Visualize calm. Close your eyes and imagine yourself in those exact moments, repeating your new responses with confidence. Do this before your next flight—you'll be surprised at how prepared you feel when those situations actually happen.

4. Choose your anchor. Pick one short phrase (max 10 words) that brings you back to calm.

Example: "Power is not danger; the plane is doing its job."

Repeat your anchor each time you exhale. Over time, your brain will connect the phrase directly with calm, making it your go-to tool in the air.

KEY TAKEAWAY

Fear of flying is not a life sentence. With awareness, visualization, breathing, grounding, and gradual exposure, you can retrain your brain. The more you practice, the more automatic these responses become—until calm becomes your new default.

Remember this: Every small victory counts. Each time you sit with your fear and use these tools, you're rewriting the script in your mind—from one of panic to one of freedom.

You now have the essential tools—awareness, visualization, breathing, grounding, and gradual exposure. They're simple, but they work. The next step is learning when to use them. In the following chapter, we'll build your personal Quick Emotional Response Kit (QERK), so you know exactly how to apply these strategies before the flight, at the airport, during turbulence, and after landing.

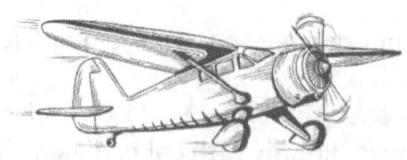

CHAPTER 7

THE QUICK EMOTIONAL RESPONSE KIT (QERK)

When I step into a cockpit, one of the first things I check is the QRH—the Quick Reference Handbook. It's a pilot's emergency playbook: short, clear checklists for every possible situation. Why? Because in moments of stress, nobody remembers a manual. You need something immediate, practical, and proven.

That's exactly what I've created for you here: the Quick Emotional Response Kit (QERK).

Think of it as your own QRH for the mind. It's not about learning new techniques—you already have them from the previous chapter. Instead, this is about knowing when and how to use them, step by step, throughout your journey.

The QERK is your pocket manual for calm: before the flight, at the airport, during turbulence, and even after landing.

BEFORE THE FLIGHT: PREPARATION AND CALM

Fear of flying often starts long before boarding. The "what if" thoughts creep in days—or even weeks—before a trip. Here's how to take control early:

1. **ANTICIPATE THE FEAR, DON'T FIGHT IT.**

Notice when your mind starts rehearsing disaster scenarios. Label it: "This is my scriptwriter at work, not reality."

2. **VISUALIZATION.**

Close your eyes and picture yourself walking calmly onto the airplane. Imagine buckling your seatbelt, smiling, breathing slowly. See yourself in control—it's mental rehearsal for success.

3. **BOX BREATHING 4×4.**

Inhale for 4, hold for 4, exhale for 4, hold for 4. Do this for two minutes before leaving home. It resets your nervous system.

Key reminder: Don't wait for the airport—start calming your mind now.

AT THE AIRPORT: BOARDING WITHOUT STRESS

Airports can feel chaotic—crowds, announcements, security checks—perfect conditions for anxiety to flare up. But with a few simple tools, you can take back control:

1. Seat choice

- Choose an aisle seat if you like the freedom to move.

- Choose a wing seat if you want less sensation of movement.

2. Hydrate wisely

Skip coffee or alcohol before flying. Both dehydrate and amplify anxiety. Water is your best ally.

3. Reset ritual

Set a playlist you enjoy and pair it with slow breathing every 15 minutes. This keeps your nervous system steady.

4. Step-out option

If the gate area feels overwhelming, step away for 3–5 minutes. Anxiety always rises and falls—let it pass instead of fighting it.

5. Ground yourself

Try the 5–4–3–2–1 technique while you wait:

- 5 things you see

- 4 things you touch

- 3 things you hear

- 2 things you smell

- 1 thing you taste

This shifts your focus from "what if" to "what is."

6. Reframe boarding

When you hear the boarding call, don't think "trap." Think:

> "This is the gateway to my destination, to my why."

7. Mini exposure

If the gate anxiety spikes, step out briefly. By feeling it and returning, you're teaching your brain: "I can handle this."

8. Ask for support

If you need extra reassurance, simply tell a flight attendant:

> "Hi, flying makes me a little nervous. I'm fine, but it helps to know what to expect. Any tips if there's turbulence?"

Cabin crew hear this often. Their calm, practical answers usually help more than you imagine.

DURING THE FLIGHT: MANAGING TURBULENCE, NOISES, AND UNKNOWNS

This is the heart of the QERK. Here's your inflight quick reference:

- ↳ Panic Reset (60 seconds)
- ↳ Long exhale (6–8 seconds).
- ↳ Box Breathing 4×4 (four cycles).
- ↳ Label: "This is anxiety, not danger."

↳ Repeat your anchor phrase.

↳ Do a micro-action: sip water or name 5 objects around you.

↳ If the wave comes back, repeat. Anxiety always rises, peaks, and drops.

1. TAKEOFF

↳ What you feel: acceleration, vibrations, noise.

↳ What to do: slow breathing + repeat: "This is power, not danger."

↳ Tip: grip the armrest loosely. Holding tight tells your brain it's unsafe.

↳ Self-brief (10 seconds):

"Noise and vibration = power. Engines quieter after climb = normal. If it shakes, I stay buckled and breathe. I've got this."

2. TURBULENCE

↳ What you feel: bumps, seatbelt sign, drinks shaking.

↳ What to do: visualize the gelatin analogy (the airplane moving inside, never falling out). Sip water slowly—it proves stability to your brain.

↳ Phrase: "Uncomfortable doesn't mean unsafe."

3. STRANGE NOISES

↳ What you hear: thumps, whirs, hums.

↳ What to do: label them: "systems at work." Say to yourself: "If it were danger, the crew wouldn't be calmly serving coffee."

4. THE SEATBELT SIGN

↳ What it means: safety precaution, not emergency.

↳ Your response: smile and think: "This is the lawyer light. It protects me."

LANDING AND AFTER THE FLIGHT: REFLECTION AND

REINFORCEMENT

As the airplane descends, you may notice:

- ↳ Ears popping (normal pressurization change).
- ↳ More noises (flaps, gear).
- ↳ Stronger sensations (descent angle, braking).

These aren't "final dangers"—they're simply signs of arrival. The airplane is doing exactly what it's designed to do.

Once you're on the ground, don't rush to forget the experience. Take two minutes to reflect:

- ↳ What worked for me today?
- ↳ When did I feel calm?
- ↳ What tools did I use successfully?

This short reflection is the key point. It transforms every flight from "just surviving" into actual training for confidence. With each trip, you're not only reaching a destination—you're building a new mindset that makes the next flight easier.

REINFORCE & REWARD

Write down three things you handled well. Then give yourself a small reward (a favorite coffee, a walk, a call to someone). Your brain learns fastest through positive reinforcement—celebrate every landing.

KEY TAKEAWAY

The QERK is your checklist for calm. You don't need to remember every detail—just the sequence:

- ↳ Before flight: prepare your mind.
- ↳ At the airport: ground yourself.
- ↳ During flight: breathe, label, reframe.
- ↳ After landing: reflect and reinforce.

Fear thrives in chaos. Calm thrives in structure. With your Quick Emotional Response Kit, you'll never be unprepared again.

You don't need to eliminate fear—you only need a checklist. And now, you have one.

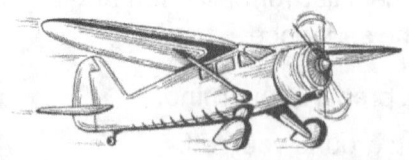

Pre-Flight Checklist

☑ Boarding Completed

☑ Understand Fear

☑ See Through the Eyes of a Pilot

☑ Take Back Control

☐ Transform Fear into Confidence

ADDITIONAL TOOLS ONBOARD

? FAQ: Real Questions from Passengers

🕐 10-Minute Pre-Flight Routine

🧠 Emotional Response Kit (QERK)

📜 Calm Scripts for Flight

PART IV
TRANSFORMATION

CHAPTER 8

YOUR WHY: THE REASON STRONGER THAN FEAR

Every passenger I've met who overcame fear of flying had one thing in common: they found a reason bigger than the fear itself.

Because fear doesn't simply disappear—it gets overpowered.

When your "why" is clear, flying stops being a threat and becomes a bridge: the path to something meaningful.

FINDING A BIGGER PURPOSE TO FLY

Ask yourself this simple question:

"Why do I want to fly?"

Not in general—but you personally.

- ↳ Maybe it's to visit your grandchildren without missing the best years of their lives.
- ↳ Maybe it's to see places you've dreamed about since childhood.
- ↳ Maybe it's to take the job that will change your career.
- ↳ Or maybe it's simply to stop saying no to life.

Fear says: "Stay here—it's safer."

Your Why says: "Go there—it matters."

Once you anchor to that bigger reason, the bumps, noises, and unknowns lose power. They're no longer walls—they're small steps on the way to something you deeply want.

STORIES OF READERS WHO TRANSFORMED THEIR FEAR

When my first book on overcoming the fear of flying was published,

I began receiving messages from readers who had put the techniques into practice.

Their experiences are proof that fear doesn't define you—it can be reshaped.

↳ •A young man in his mid-twenties. He had always avoided flying, never once crossing the Atlantic because the idea felt unbearable. After reading the book, he finally boarded a flight to New York. The experience gave him confidence, and months later, he did it again—this time flying to Mexico for vacation. Two long journeys in one year, after years of avoidance.

↳ •A reader from Denver. She described her first flight after reading the book as a real test: heavy turbulence, a technical issue, and even a deplaning. In the past, this chain of events would have been overwhelming. Instead, she surprised herself. She stayed grounded, managed her fear, and completed the journey. Later, she wrote to thank me, saying: "I couldn't have done it before. This time, I was ready."

↳ •A frequent business traveler. He admitted that fear still shows up on many flights. But after applying the strategies in this book, he now feels in control. Instead of canceling trips or suffering in silence, he travels with a calm mind, able to focus on his work and life beyond the airplane.

↳ •An older woman. She had never flown in her life because of fear. But after reading the book, something changed: she now feels prepared and motivated. Even without stepping onto a plane yet, her mindset is different. She told me: "For the first time, I'm not dreading it—I'm looking forward to it." Sometimes, the biggest transformation begins in the mind, before the first takeoff.

Every story is different—but the theme is the same. Their "Why" was stronger than fear.

These aren't extraordinary people—they're ordinary passengers who chose to anchor to their "Why". And if they can do it, so can you.

TURNING FLIGHTS INTO OPPORTUNITIES, NOT THREATS

Here's the real breakthrough: flying doesn't have to be something you endure. It can be something you use. Every flight is a training ground—a chance to practice your tools, to prove to yourself that you are stronger than your fear.

- What if, instead of seeing turbulence as a threat, you saw it as a chance to practice calm breathing?

- What if, instead of dreading the engine sounds, you used them as reminders that the systems are working exactly as designed?

- What if, instead of walking off the plane with relief, you walked off with pride—knowing you grew stronger in the process?

This is transformation: fear turning into growth, anxiety turning into opportunity, the airplane turning from a cage into a classroom of freedom.

PRACTICAL EXERCISE – DISCOVER YOUR WHY

Take a notebook and write:

What's my personal reason to fly? (family, career, adventure, freedom)

What do I lose if I let fear decide? (missed moments, regrets, limits)

What do I gain when I face it? (connection, opportunity, pride)

Circle the one that hits you hardest. That's your Why.

Before your next flight, read it. Say it out loud. Carry it with you like a compass.

KEY TAKEAWAY

Fear doesn't vanish by itself. But it gets smaller when it collides with something bigger.

Your Why is that bigger thing.

Every time you fly, don't focus on what you fear—focus on what you're flying toward.

That's how fear turns into freedom.

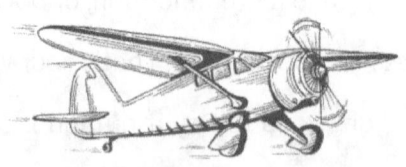

CHAPTER 9

THE PATH FORWARD: CONFIDENCE FOR A LIFETIME

Overcoming the fear of flying isn't about one flight—it's about building confidence that lasts a lifetime. You've now learned the tools, the strategies, and even the stories of others who've walked this path. The next step is making sure the progress sticks, so that flying becomes part of your freedom—not your prison.

HOW TO MAINTAIN PROGRESS AND AVOID SETBACKS

Progress isn't a straight line. Some flights will feel easier, others may trigger old fears. That's normal. The difference now is that you have the skills to handle it.

Think of setbacks as turbulence. They may shake you, but they don't stop you from moving forward.

HERE'S HOW TO STAY ON TRACK

- •Keep practicing. Even on flights that feel calm, rehearse your breathing, grounding, and visualization. Skills stay sharp when you use them.
- •Reflect, don't judge. If fear shows up again, don't call it failure. Write down what triggered it, which tool you used, and what worked. This is learning, not losing.
- •Celebrate the wins. Every flight completed, every calm moment reclaimed, is progress. Reward yourself—it reinforces your brain to keep going.

BUILDING EMPOWERING BELIEFS DAILY

Your thoughts shape your flying experience long before you step on the plane. That's why building daily empowering beliefs matters.

HERE ARE THREE SIMPLE PRACTICES:

↳ Morning mantra. Start your day with a phrase like:

"I can handle what comes my way. Fear is just noise—I decide the meaning."

↳ Visualization habit. Spend two minutes imagining yourself calm on a flight. Small doses add up.

↳ Anchor to success. Recall your calmest flight or your proudest moment of facing fear. Relive it. Let your body feel that memory.

Little by little, these habits shift your identity. You're no longer "someone afraid of flying"—you're "someone who can fly."

MAKING FLYING PART OF YOUR FREEDOM, NOT YOUR PRISON

The ultimate goal isn't just to fly—it's to reclaim your freedom. Flying is the bridge to your dreams, your family, your adventures.

When you step onto an airplane, remind yourself:

↳ • This isn't punishment—it's possibility.

↳ • This isn't a cage—it's a door to the world.

↳ • This isn't about surviving—it's about living.

Reframing flying this way makes every trip an act of empowerment, not fear.

PRACTICAL EXERCISE – YOUR CONFIDENCE CONTRACT

Write a short "contract" with yourself that includes:

↳ My Why – the reason I choose to fly (family, freedom, opportunities).

↳ My Tools – the techniques I commit to using (breathing, grounding, visualization, reflection).

↳ My Promise – "I will not let fear decide for me. Every flight I take is proof that courage grows when I use my tools."

Keep it in your wallet or phone. Read it before every flight. This isn't just paper—it's a commitment to freedom and a reminder that you're in charge, not fear.

KEY TAKEAWAY

Fear may knock on the door from time to time—but now, you don't have to let it in.

Confidence isn't the absence of fear. It's the knowledge that you can handle it.

Every flight from now on is more than a journey from point A to point B. It's proof that you are stronger than your fear, and that your freedom is greater than your limits.

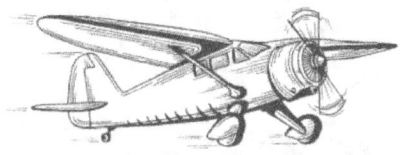

Pre-Flight Checklist

☑ <u>Boarding Completed</u>

☑ <u>Understand Fear</u>

☑ <u>See Through the Eyes of a Pilot</u>

☑ <u>Take Back Control</u>

☑ <u>Transform Fear into Confidence</u>

ADDITIONAL TOOLS ONBOARD

? FAQ: Real Questions from Passengers

🕐 10-Minute Pre-Flight Routine

🧠 Emotional Response Kit (QERK)

📋 Calm Scripts for Flight

FAQ
Frequently Asked Questions from My Passengers

Over the years, I've had countless conversations with passengers—some curious, some anxious, others simply wanting reassurance. Many of the same questions come up again and again, both in the cockpit and during flights.

This section gathers the most common ones, with the same honest answers I've shared thousands of times. My goal is simple: to give you clarity where there's doubt, and calm where there's fear.

1. SAFETY AND HOW AIRPLANES WORK

WHAT HAPPENS IF BOTH ENGINES FAIL?

First, let me calm your mind: the chance of this happening is so tiny that it's almost science fiction. Think about your house: how often do two light bulbs burn out at the exact same time? Almost never. Airplane engines are even more reliable than your light bulbs.

Now, let's play with the "what if." Modern airplanes are designed to glide. That means that even without engines, the plane does not fall from the sky—it keeps flying, like a huge glider. Our first action as pilots would be to restart the engines (we train this constantly). If that didn't work, we'd still have time and distance to find a safe place to land.

So no, the sky doesn't "switch off." The airplane keeps flying.

CAN AN AIRPLANE FLY WITH ONLY ONE ENGINE?

Yes, perfectly. In fact, every route we fly is planned knowing that if one engine failed, the plane could continue safely. I've flown on one engine in training, and the plane feels strong and controllable. It can even keep its altitude.

WHAT IF THE PILOT GETS SICK DURING THE FLIGHT?

This is what we call "pilot incapacitation." We train for it just like we train for engine failures. If one pilot feels unwell, the other takes full control. The airplane is designed to be flown by one pilot if necessary. And in most cases, we'd simply land at the nearest airport to get medical help.

WHAT IF LIGHTNING STRIKES THE PLANE?

It has happened to me several times in my career. The truth? Nothing dramatic. A lightning strike usually enters from one point, exits from another, and continues its path. The airplane is designed like a Faraday cage, which means the electricity stays outside, not inside the cabin. The only inconvenience is that once on the ground, the aircraft needs a detailed inspection before the next flight.

CAN SUCH A HEAVY AIRPLANE REALLY TAKE OFF FROM A SHORT RUNWAY?

If it takes off, it's because it can. Period. Before every flight, calculations are made considering weight, weather, runway length, and more. If those numbers don't work, we don't take off. So if you're sitting in a plane that's accelerating on a runway, it's because the math is already in your favor.

WHAT IF THERE'S AN EMERGENCY AND NO AIRPORT NEARBY?

We always have a plan. Long before the engines start, we check alternate airports, fuel reserves, and emergency scenarios. Even in remote areas, regulations require us to carry extra fuel so we always have options. Emergencies are rare, but the preparation for them is constant.

CAN SOMEONE OPEN THE DOOR DURING THE FLIGHT?

No. Not even close. Airplane doors work like giant plugs. The pressure inside pushes them tightly into the frame, making them impossible to open at cruising altitude. Imagine trying to pull a cork out of a bottle of champagne while it's still under pressure— it won't happen.

CAN STRONG WINDS PUSH THE AIRPLANE DANGEROUSLY?

No. The airplane moves with the wind like a balloon drifting in a stream, but we always remain in control of direction and speed. What passengers might feel as "being pushed around" is just turbulence, which is uncomfortable but not unsafe.

WHAT SOUNDS MEAN SOMETHING IS WRONG, AND WHICH ARE NORMAL?

Airplanes make many sounds—hydraulic pumps, wing flaps, landing gear, even furniture settling. To a pilot, almost all of them are normal. When something truly requires our attention, the airplane doesn't whisper—it shouts. We get alarms, lights, and clear warnings.

DO PILOTS HEAR ALARMS WHEN SOMETHING FAILS?

Yes. Just like your car shows a red oil light or a beep when you forget the seatbelt, airplanes have systems that alert us with sounds and lights. In fact, the system is so advanced that sometimes it alerts us before there's even a real problem.

2. TURBULENCE AND WEATHER

CAN TURBULENCE FLIP AN AIRPLANE?

No. Turbulence can shake, bump, and make you feel like you're on a roller coaster, but it cannot flip an airplane. Imagine an airplane suspended in a bowl of gelatin. Shake the bowl and the airplane wiggles—but it never falls out.

CAN PILOTS PREDICT OR AVOID TURBULENCE?

Yes, most of the time. We don't have a "turbulence radar," but we do have detailed weather reports, flight planning tools, and other pilots ahead of us sharing real-time updates. If turbulence is expected, we can often avoid it by changing altitude or route.

WHAT DO PILOTS DO WHEN THE WEATHER IS VERY BAD?

We don't take risks. If weather is outside safe limits, the flight doesn't leave. Period. Sometimes, what passengers call "bad weather" (like rain in London) is nothing to us. But if there's a hurricane or severe storm, flights are delayed or canceled. Safety always wins over schedules.

WHY DOES THE AIRPLANE MOVE MORE WHEN LANDING?

Close to the ground, the air is more unstable because it flows over buildings, mountains, or hot surfaces. That makes landings sometimes bumpy. But remember: airplanes are designed to handle these conditions, and pilots train hundreds of times for landings in all kinds of wind.

3. PASSENGER EXPERIENCE

WHY DO THE ENGINES SOMETIMES SOUND LOUDER, THEN QUIETER?

It's the same as your car on a hill. More power, louder sound. Less power, quieter sound. During takeoff, we demand maximum power. In cruise, less is needed. That's all you're hearing—the engine working as it should.

WHAT ARE THOSE BANGS AND KNOCKS DURING THE FLIGHT?

Airplanes are full of moving parts—flaps, landing gear, hydraulic pumps. Add to that the cabin fittings shifting slightly. Most noises are just the sound of a machine working. If there were a real problem, we'd know instantly.

WHY DO THE WINGS BEND SO MUCH IN TURBULENCE?

Because they're supposed to. Flexibility is strength. Think of a palm tree in the wind—it bends instead of breaking. Modern wings, like those on the Boeing 787, can bend dramatically without risk.

WHY DOES IT SOMETIMES FEEL LIKE THE AIRPLANE SUDDENLY DROPS?

It's an illusion. The plane might move a few feet down in turbulence, but inside, it feels like an elevator dropping. Next time, put a glass of water on your tray. Watch how little it moves compared to how much your body feels it.

WHY ARE CABIN LIGHTS DIMMED FOR TAKEOFF AND LANDING?

It's a safety precaution. At night, your eyes need about 30 minutes to adapt to darkness. By dimming the lights, your vision adjusts so that if there were an emergency evacuation, you'd already see better outside.

WHAT DOES THE SEATBELT SIGN REALLY MEAN?

Exactly what it says: put it on. Turbulence can appear suddenly, and the seatbelt keeps you safely in place. It's the simplest and most effective safety measure on board.

4. HEALTH AND ANXIETY

SHOULD I TAKE PILLS OR ALCOHOL BEFORE FLYING?

No. Pills and alcohol only mask fear, and often make anxiety worse in the long run. The real solution is understanding and practicing the tools you'll find in this book.

WHAT CAN I DO IF I HAVE A PANIC ATTACK ON THE PLANE?

That's exactly why I've filled this book with practical techniques. Breathing exercises, grounding tools, and scripts are your best allies. The key is preparation—don't wait until panic arrives.

DO MEDITATION OR BREATHING REALLY WORK DURING A FLIGHT?

Yes, but only if you've practiced before. Just like you wouldn't run a marathon without training, you can't expect to master meditation on your first try in the air. The more you practice on the ground, the more effective it becomes in the sky.

WHAT IF I'M CLAUSTROPHOBIC OR AFRAID OF NOT BEING ABLE TO GET OUT?

That fear is common, and it comes from the mind creating "what if" stories. The truth: airplanes are designed with multiple exits and clear procedures. The sense of being trapped is an illusion. The techniques in this book will help you redirect that thought.

WHAT IF I PANIC AND WANT TO GET OFF THE PLANE?

Of course, you can't leave mid-flight. That's why it's important to recognize panic early and use the tools I give you here—breathing, reframing, grounding. Panic rises fast, but it also falls fast when you don't fuel it.

5. GENERAL QUESTIONS

HOW COMMON IS FEAR OF FLYING?

More common than you think. About 1 in 3 passengers feels anxiety about flying. So if you feel nervous, remember: you're not strange, you're not broken—you're human.

CAN I REALLY OVERCOME IT, OR WILL I JUST LEARN TO LIVE WITH IT?

You can absolutely overcome it. The key is having a strong reason—your "why." I've seen people go from panic attacks to becoming pilots themselves. If your motivation is strong enough, progress is possible.

HOW LONG DOES IT TAKE TO LOSE THE FEAR?

That depends on you. Some people feel a big change after one flight using these tools. Others need several. Like any skill, the more you practice, the faster you progress.

HOW DO PILOTS STAY CALM ALL THE TIME?

Training and repetition. We prepare for every possible situation again and again until it becomes routine. You may not fly every day, but you can "train your brain" daily with visualization and mental practice—just like elite athletes do.

WHY DO THEY SAY FLYING IS THE SAFEST TRANSPORT?

Because it is. Aviation is one of the most regulated industries in the world. Every incident leads to improvements, every detail is studied, and the result is clear: statistically, flying is the safest way to travel.

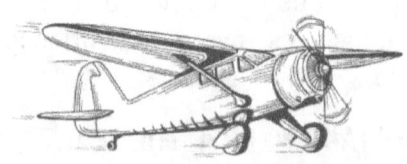

Resources and Next Steps

Finishing this book is not the end of your journey—it's the beginning of a new chapter in your freedom to fly. If you want to keep building confidence and stay connected, here are the next steps:

1. AUTHOR PAGE

Visit www.ronbengoechea.com to find more resources, updates, and ways to continue this journey.

2. STAY IN TOUCH

If you'd like to share your story, ask a question, or simply let me know how this book has helped you, you can reach me directly:

fly@ronbengoechea.com

I personally read every message—I'd love to hear from you.

3. UPCOMING BOOK: 365 LETTERS AGAINST FEAR

I'm currently writing my third book, 365 Letters Against Fear. It will be a collection of daily letters—one for each day of the year—designed to help you retrain your mind and overcome fear step by step.

If you'd like to receive a preview or be notified when it's released, just send me an email. I'll be glad to keep you updated.

4. KEEP PRACTICING YOUR TOOLS

Remember, you already have the essentials:

↳ Your Why (Chapter 8)

↳ Your Quick Emotional Response Kit (Chapter 7)

↳ Your Confidence Contract (Chapter 9)

↳ The 10-Minutes Pre-Flight Poutine (Appendix C)

Review them before each flight. Each time you fly, you're not just traveling—you're proving to yourself that fear no longer controls you.

The journey doesn't stop here. Stay connected, keep practicing, and remember: you are stronger than your fear.

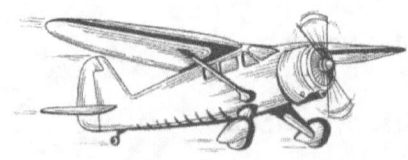

CLOSING

FINAL REFLECTION: FLYING AS A METAPHOR FOR LIFE

Overcoming the fear of flying is not just about airplanes—it's about life itself. Each page you've read, each exercise you've practiced, has been a step toward reclaiming your freedom.

I am deeply grateful that you trusted me to be your captain on this journey. Writing this book was my way of sharing what I've seen from the cockpit, but the real courage came from you—choosing to face your fear and refusing to let it define your life.

Now, your story doesn't end here. Every time you board an airplane, you're not just traveling to a destination—you're proving to yourself that growth is possible, that calm can replace panic, and that freedom is stronger than fear.

My wish for you is simple: that flying becomes a bridge, not a barrier. That every takeoff reminds you of new beginnings, every landing of safe arrivals, and every flight of your own inner strength.

And remember this: you are no longer just a passenger. From now on, you are a Travelnauta—a traveler of skies and of life, someone who dares to move forward with courage and purpose.

Keep navigating your skies. Your freedom has just taken off.

With gratitude,

From the Flight Deck,
Ronald Bengoechea

Acknowledgements

First, to you—the reader. You are the heart of this book. Each page exists because of your trust, your courage, and your willingness to face the sky with me. Without you, there would be no reason to write.

To my wife, Jenny—thank you for walking every step of this journey with me. In this second edition, I am even more aware that none of this would be possible without your strength, patience, and encouragement. You are my safe harbor.

To my daughter, Sofía—in the first version, I wanted this book to be something you could read one day and use as a guide. In this second version, I dedicate it to the person you are becoming. May these words remind you not only that courage is stronger than fear, but also that resilience, curiosity, and kindness will take you even further than any airplane ever could. I am proud of the person you are and the one you are becoming.

And finally, to every new Travelnauta who takes these ideas into their own life: thank you. Your transformation is the true fuel of this project. Every story you share, every fear you face, keeps me inspired to keep flying this mission with you.

With gratitude and hope for your journeys ahead,

Ronald Bengoechea

Appendix A - Emotional Response Kit

QERK – QUICK EMOTIONAL RESPONSE KIT

Your pocket manual for calm.

Before the Flight

- ↳ Label fear: "Scriptwriter, not reality."
- ↳ Visualize: calm boarding, seatbelt on, breathing slow.
- ↳ Box Breathing 4×4 for 2 minutes.

AT THE AIRPORT

- ↳ Grounding 5–4–3–2–1: see, touch, hear, smell, taste.
- ↳ Hydrate (skip coffee/alcohol).
- ↳ Reset ritual: playlist + slow breath every 15 min.
- ↳ Reframe: "This is my gateway to my why."
- ↳ If overwhelmed: step out 3–5 minutes, then return.

DURING THE FLIGHT

PANIC RESET (60 SEC):

- ↳ Long exhale (6–8s)
- ↳ Box Breathing 4×4, (4 cycles)

Label: "This is anxiety, not danger."

Anchor phrase (your choice)

Micro-action: sip water, name 5 objects

TAKEOFF SELF-BRIEF (10 SEC):

"Noise = power. Engines quieter = normal. If it shakes, I breathe. I've got this."

Turbulence: "Uncomfortable ≠ unsafe." (Gelatin analogy)

Strange noises: "Systems at work. Crew calm = I'm safe."

Seatbelt sign: "Lawyer light—it protects me."

LANDING & AFTER THE FLIGHT

↳ Pops, flaps, gear = signs of arrival, not danger.

↳ Reflect: What worked? When did I feel calm? What tools did I use?

↳ Reward yourself: celebrate every landing.

KEY REMINDER

Fear thrives in chaos. Calm thrives in structure.

With your QERK, you'll never be unprepared again.

Appendix B - Calm Scripts

CALM SCRIPTS

When fear strikes during a flight, your brain goes into survival mode. In that state, long explanations or technical reasoning don't work—your nervous system is too busy reacting. What does work is short, direct phrases that act as anchors.

These are not mystical chants. They are cognitive tools. By repeating a clear, factual statement, you're sending your brain and body a signal: "This is safe. I am in control." Psychologists call this cognitive reframing—replacing catastrophic thoughts with truths that calm your nervous system.

Think of them as your personal checklist for the mind, just like pilots use short checklists in the cockpit. Simple, direct, effective.

CALM SCRIPTS COLLECTION

↳ "Power means safety, not danger."
↳ "Uncomfortable ≠ unsafe."
↳ "I breathe; the airplane keeps me safe."
↳ "Noise is systems working, not problems."
↳ "The crew is calm, so I am safe."
↳ "Turbulence is movement, not threat."
↳ "Wings bend because they're strong."
↳ "This airplane is built for more than this."
↳ "Fear is a story, not reality."
↳ "Every bump proves the plane is working."

HOW TO USE THEM

- ↪ Choose 2 or 3 phrases that feel natural to you.
- ↪ Practice them before your flight—say them out loud or write them down.
- ↪ Use them in the moment: during turbulence, takeoff, or whenever fear rises, repeat your chosen phrase slowly with each breath.
- ↪ Combine with breathing: Inhale... repeat the first half. Exhale... repeat the second half.

EXAMPLE:

Inhale: "I breathe..."

Exhale: "...the airplane keeps me safe."

This pairing of calm words and calm breathing teaches your nervous system that it can relax—even in the middle of turbulence.

Appendix C - Pre-Flight Routine

THE 10-MINUTE PRE-FLIGHT ROUTINE

Preparation is 50% of calm. Just like pilots follow a checklist before flying, you can follow your own. Print it, save it on your phone, or keep it in your bag. Use it every time before boarding.

MINUTE 1–2: BREATHING START-UP

↳ Do four cycles of 4x4 breathing (inhale 4 – hold 4 – exhale 4 – hold 4).

↳ Tell your nervous system: "I am safe."

MINUTE 3: MENTAL ANCHOR

↳ Repeat your calming phrase, for example:
  ↳ "Inhale calm, exhale tension."
  ↳ "I am in control of my response."

MINUTE 4–5: QUICK VISUALIZATION

↳ Imagine yourself walking calmly toward the plane.

↳ See yourself seated, breathing deeply.

↳ Feel takeoff as pure power, not danger.

↳ Picture yourself enjoying the journey.

MINUTE 6–7: GROUNDING IN THE PRESENT

↳ 5 things you see.

↳ 4 things you can touch.

↳ 3 sounds you hear.

- ↳ 2 scents you notice.
- ↳ 1 taste in your mouth.

MINUTE 8: PHYSICAL RESET

- ↳ Relax shoulders, jaw, and hands.
- ↳ Drink a sip of water.
- ↳ Stretch neck and back gently.

MINUTE 9: REVIEW YOUR "WHY"

- ↳ Read your written motivation: visiting family, vacation, opportunity.
- ↳ Remind yourself: "This is why I choose to fly."

MINUTE 10: MENTAL CONTRACT

- ↳ Say to yourself:

"I'm ready. I know what I feel, I know what happens in my body, and I know the airplane is designed to keep me safe. I don't need to fight fear—I just travel with it."

RESULT

In 10 minutes, you move from reactive to prepared. Just like a pilot, you start your flight with confidence switched on.